MENOPAUSE MADE

Kendra Sundquist, who holds a Master's degree in Health Science Education, is a nursing educator who has had 15 years' experience as a practitioner in the field of sexual and reproductive health.

MENOPAUSE MADE EASY

KENDRA SUNDQUIST

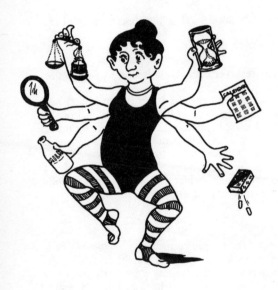

ROBINSON
London

Robinson Publishing Ltd
7 Kensington Church Court
London W8 4SP

First published in Great Britain by
Robinson Publishing Ltd 1995

Published in Australia by
Gore & Osment Publications Pty Ltd

Copyright © Kendra Sundquist 1992

Copyright © Gore & Osment Publications Pty Ltd

ISBN 1–85487–383–0

A copy of the British Library Cataloguing in Publication
Data is available from the British Library

Note
This book is not a substitute for your doctor's or health
professional's advice, and the publishers and author
cannot accept liability for any injury or loss to any
person acting or refraining from action as a result of
the material in this book. Before commencing any
health treatment, always consult your doctor.

Printed and bound in Great Britain

Contents

Introduction

Are you one of the many women who worry about menopause? Well you can stop worrying about it, right now. No one has ever died from the menopause. Much of the anxiety about menopause is caused by not knowing what to expect. This book will help you to understand what is happening to your body and why it is happening. As a result, you will feel less anxious and more in control. You will also learn what you can do to help yourself and where to go if you need outside help.

Change of any kind takes a bit of getting used to. 'Change of Life' can be, and should be, a change for the better. Menopause comes at the same time as middle age, a time when there are many changes and adjustments to make. Nothing in life ever stays the same.

It's a bit like walking up stairs: even if you stayed on the same step forever, and never went any further, the scene around you would go on changing.

A century ago, women only lived to about 50 years of age. Today, you can expect to live 30 years or so longer. This means you have a lot of living to do after menopause; a third of your life, in fact. Yes, there is certainly life after menopause!

Look on menopause as the beginning of a new phase in your life, not an ending. In fact, it can be the most creative time of your life, offering you new freedom to develop and pursue your own interests.

Most importantly, you will still be the same *you* as you were before menopause.

Chapter I
What's Going to Happen to Me?

There are many rumours, myths and tall stories about menopause and the horrors that women have to endure. Let's take a closer look at some of these and sort out the fact from the fiction.

MENOPAUSE FACTS

The word 'menopause' literally means the time when your periods cease permanently.

- It is a natural process for all women, a biological change that usually occurs between the ages of 45 to 55 years, with the average at about 51 to 52 years. Of course there is a small percentage of women who will experience menopause before 45 years and others who will have a later menopause, after the age of 55.

- Menopause means the end of your reproductive years. In other words, you will no longer be able to have a baby.

- The experience of menopause will be different for each individual and symptoms will vary from woman to woman. Most symptoms that surround menopause or develop after it are caused by a lack of hormones. The most common symptoms that women experience are: hot flushes, sweating, mood changes, anxiety, depression, anger, dry or sore vagina, palpitations, poor sleep, aches and pains, more frequent headaches, poor memory, bladder problems, dry skin, itching or burning skin, loss of interest in sex.

  The majority of women will experience only a few symptoms.

  Whether a woman decides to seek help or chooses to ignore the symptoms, will depend how much she is bothered by them.

  A small percentage of women will have no symptoms at all – their periods will simply stop and that's it. Another small percentage will have symptoms that really trouble them and they will need to seek help.

MENOPAUSE MYTHS

'Irritable', 'unattractive', 'neurotic', 'hard to live with' – how often have you heard these things said about women at menopause? Many of these negative stereotypes come from advertisements, newspapers, magazines and television. It's no wonder that women lose confidence in themselves in mid-life. Other common misconceptions are:

- You have some kind of illness or disease.
- Menopause is a sign you are old.
- Some women go crazy. This one is a relic from centuries ago when women were locked up in mental institutions at menopause.
- You will no longer feel like having sex and no one will find you sexually attractive.
- You will get fat and lose your looks.
- You will not be able to cope.

These stories, and others like them, are just not true – so don't believe a word of them.

Sixty or 70 years ago, menopause was never talked about. It wasn't even mentioned in any of the medical journals. Today, women and men are living much longer than ever before. In fact, women outlive men by about 6 or 7 years. By the year 2050, women will probably live to be at least 95. Because of this, menopause has suddenly become big business. Doctors, drug companies, the media and governments are all now very interested in every aspect of menopause and ageing.

Some experts, usually doctors, view menopause as a disease that must be treated; others see it as a more natural process. If even the experts can't agree, no wonder we women are confused! One expert says, 'Menopause is a sex-linked, female-dominant, endocrine deficiency disease which should be investigated and managed in a careful way for the rest of a woman's life'. Sounds like a real health hazard, doesn't it? It's a wonder that any of us survive!

The purpose of this book is to help you take control of your own menopause. One of the best things about knowing the facts is that you can then make your own decisions about what is best for you. If you do have symptoms, you will be better able to discuss them with your doctor, because you will know what questions to ask.

STAGES OF MENOPAUSE

Strictly speaking, menopause refers to the time when menstruation ceases. You can only really be sure that this has happened when you have gone for twelve months without a period.

Q. *When will this happen?*
A. For most women, menopause will occur between the ages of 45 and 55. If it occurs before the age of 40, it is called a premature menopause. Relatively few women experience menopause before the age of 40 or after 55.

Q. *If I started menstruating early, will I have an early menopause?*
A. Whether you started menstruating at an early age or much later, doesn't seem to make any difference to the age at which you will experience the menopause. However, menopause does seem to occur at a similar age in

mothers and their daughters. If you have sisters, then it is likely that you and they will experience menopause at a similar age.

Q. *What is the climacteric or peri-menopause?*
A. These are the medical terms that refer to the years before and after the menopause. 'Climacteric' comes from a Greek word meaning 'step on a ladder', because it marks the beginning of a new phase in your life.

During puberty, your body goes through a 'winding up' process, with many changes occurring before menstruation begins. In the climacteric stage, your body is also changing as part of the 'winding down' process of your reproductive function. Both puberty and the climacteric represent the beginning and ending of a different stage of your life.

What happens during this stage will vary from woman to woman. You may notice changes in your periods. They may become more frequent or more infrequent. Blood flow may be different. It can either be lighter and more watery or it can be very heavy, with clots.

You may also experience mood changes or physical symptoms, such as hot flushes, sweating, weight-gain and sleep problems.

Q. *What causes the symptoms?*
A. During this winding down process, the production of your female hormones is dropping. This happens in an irregular way. You will have sudden bursts of high and low levels of

hormone production, causing symptoms, such as hot flushes, sweating and mood changes. It can take months or even years for your body to adjust to these changes.

Q. *Why does menopause occur?*
A. When you were born you had about 2 million follicles, or egg-forming cells, in your ovaries. By the time you reached puberty, there were only about 500,000: the rest had died. From then on, one or two of these egg cells ripened during each menstrual cycle and others died.

At menopause, you will have only about 8,000 of these egg cells left. Gradually, your ovaries will stop releasing an egg each month and the remaining egg cells will just disappear.

Your ovaries also produce two hormones: oestrogen and progesterone. After menopause, the production of these hormones will slow down, affecting your periods and causing other noticeable changes.

ARTIFICIAL MENOPAUSE

Menopause that does not occur naturally is described as artificial. It can happen because of:

Surgery where both ovaries are removed. There can be a number of reasons why such surgery is necessary:

Endometriosis, a condition in which the lining of the uterus (womb) begins to grow outside the uterus, over the ovaries and, sometimes, over the bowel as well. During the monthly period, there is also bleeding from these areas of tissue, causing severe pain.

Ovarian cysts are quite common and, in most cases, do not cause too much trouble. If they are causing problems, the cysts can be easily removed. Sometimes, if the cysts are very large, the ovaries are damaged in the process and will also need to be removed.

Cancer, such as breast cancer, can sometimes spread to other parts of the body. In this case, the ovaries are often removed because the oestrogen they produce is believed to stimulate the growth of cancer cells, if they are already present. If the ovaries themselves are cancerous, they will be removed.

Irradiation, which is sometimes used to prevent an existing cancer from spreading, can destroy the ovaries and stop them from functioning.

Chemotherapy, a special drug treatment for cancer, can also destroy the ovaries and stop them from functioning.

Q. *How will I feel after an artificial menopause?*
A. Because you will have a sudden menopause and not experience the winding down stage naturally, you may not be as well prepared, either emotionally or physically. You may have

no immediate symptoms but, on the other hand, you may experience hot flushes within a week or two of an artificial menopause. If this happens, you will need to take hormones.

Q. *What can I do about my feelings?*
A. Talk to your doctor about the possible consequences of any of these treatments and have an action plan ready. Be prepared to experience grief – losing any part of our body can cause a sense of loss. If you are a young woman, you may feel very sad that you will no longer be able to have a child. Each of us is likely to react differently to the situation, depending on how we view it, and what special meaning it has for us.

You may feel very angry, especially if you do not understand why your ovaries were removed. It is very important that you are able to discuss your feelings of anger and loss with someone who can help you to come to terms with them, such as your doctor or a counsellor.

IT'S TIME TO FEEL GOOD!

Feeling good about yourself at any time in your life is important – especially so at menopause. The physical symptoms you may experience are often not the main problem.

We live in a world where a lot of emphasis is placed on youth and beauty. Older women often feel at a loss, because they no longer fit this ideal image. Some women say they feel as though they are invisible and no longer regarded as a person.

Well, it's about time to shake off some of these negative attitudes towards older women. You have probably spent the last 20 or 30 years of your life worrying about everyone else – your partner, your family or your children. Well, your time has finally arrived – so go for it!

BE PREPARED

- Find out all you can about menopause.
- Talk about your concerns, don't suffer in silence.
- Find a good doctor when you need one and don't ever feel guilty about asking for help.
- Recognise that the more you stand up for what you want, the more likely you are to get it.
- Look forward to the rest of your life!

REMEMBER

- Menopause is a natural event, not a disease.

Chapter 2
'Down There': Your Body and You

Your body is a unique and fascinating machine. Most of us never really think about how our bodies work until something goes wrong. We women are unique. We experience cyclical changes in our bodies each month and are able to bear children.

The cyclical changes are caused by the action of certain glands, or organs, which produce important hormones. Hormones are like messengers which control many of our vital processes and act on nearly every living cell in our bodies.

It is very important for you to understand how hormones can affect you, particularly in regard to your menstrual cycle or monthly period. It is also important to understand how these hormones can cause changes in your body. These changes are most noticeable at puberty, during pregnancy and at menopause.

SEX HORMONES

Deep inside your head is a part of your brain (hypothalamus) and an endocrine gland (pituitary gland) which manufactures hormones. These are responsible for the changes that occur in both girls and boys around puberty.

The female sex hormones are called oestrogen and progesterone. The male sex hormones (of which testosterone is one) are called androgens. Men and women have both male and female hormones.

The ovaries produce oestrogen and progesterone as well as a small amount of testosterone. In men, testosterone is produced by the testes. The adrenal glands which sit on top of the kidneys also produce a little of both male and female hormones.

Androgens (male hormones) are responsible for the deeper voice, muscular development and more aggressive behaviour of men. To a certain extent, they also control sexual desire.

Production of sex hormones can be affected by all sorts of things, such as stress, illness and even too much or too little body fat.

After menopause, the ovaries continue to produce small amounts of oestrogen as well as testosterone. At this time, the adrenal glands take over the production of hormones from the ovaries. These are converted into oestrogen in the body fat. This is one of the reasons for the so-called middle-aged spread and is nature's way of ensuring that you have enough oestrogen. In fact, after the menopause, fatter women will age more slowly than very thin women.

From the age of about 40, your ovaries become less responsive to the pituitary hormones that control them. This makes you less fertile and reduces the amounts of ovarian hormones you produce.

UNDERSTANDING MENSTRUATION

There has always been something rather magical about blood and menstruation. Throughout history, menstruating women have been regarded as having special powers. Even in the Bible we find texts describing a menstruating woman as unclean and, moreover, everything she touched was also considered unclean. She was forbidden to have sex and was sometimes forced to live apart until after her period was finished.

Some people believed that menstruating women could ruin the crops, turn the milk sour and even cause natural disasters, such as fire or floods!

Of course, no one believes these stories today but, even so, menstruation is often seen as a sickness and the blood is often seen as unhygienic. Neither of these beliefs is true.

Menstruation is also called 'a period', 'the curse' (short for 'the curse of Eve' because of what she did to Adam in the Garden of Eden), 'the rags' and numerous other strange names. It usually begins between the ages of 12 and 14 years, but can occur as early as 9 or 10 or not until 16 or even later.

MENSTRUATION

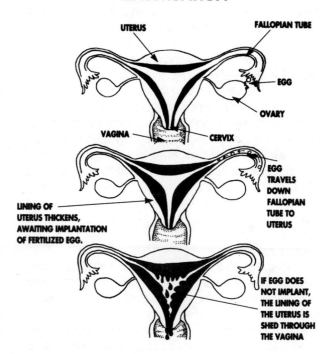

UTERUS

FALLOPIAN TUBE

EGG

OVARY

VAGINA

CERVIX

LINING OF UTERUS THICKENS, AWAITING IMPLANTATION OF FERTILIZED EGG.

EGG TRAVELS DOWN FALLOPIAN TUBE TO UTERUS

IF EGG DOES NOT IMPLANT, THE LINING OF THE UTERUS IS SHED THROUGH THE VAGINA

What is Menstruation?

Menstruation is the regular shedding of the lining of your uterus (womb). This lining is called the endometrium.

In the first part of your cycle, this lining grows and becomes thick with lots of rich blood vessels as it prepares to receive a fertilised egg.

If there is no fertilised egg (in other words if you are not pregnant) the lining stops growing and starts to break down. As it comes away, it is shed into the vagina as menstrual fluid, composed of blood, cells, mucous and bits of the lining itself. The actual cycle itself varies from woman to woman. Anywhere between 21 and 35 days is normal. The average cycle is about 27–30 days between periods.

The bleeding varies too. Some women bleed for two or three days while others bleed for five or six. The blood flow can be very light, medium or heavy. The average blood loss is between 50–80 ml. The cycle can be affected by stress, diet, illness, travel or excessive exercise.

What Happens During Menstruation?

Day 1 onwards

The first day of bleeding is Day 1. Oestrogen and progesterone are at a low level. This encourages the hypothalamus and the pituitary gland to begin producing another hormone (follicle stimulating hormone (FSH)), which in turn stimulates many of the egg follicles in the ovaries to grow. When these egg follicles grow, they produce oestrogen which is then carried by the bloodstream to the uterus (womb), where it causes the lining to thicken, ready to receive the fertilised egg. When there is enough oestrogen,

the pituitary gland releases a luteinising hormone (LH) which stops most of the other egg
follicles from developing any further but allows
one of them to develop to maturity.

Day 12 onwards
When the egg follicle is developed it is released
from the ovary. This is called ovulation. The egg
is wafted into the fallopian tube and it then
moves down towards the uterus. When the egg
is released from the ovary, it leaves behind a
scar called the corpus luteum which produces
progesterone for the next 14 days, helping to
ready the lining of the uterus for a pregnancy.

Day 15 onwards
The level of progesterone rises in the bloodstream as the lining of the uterus prepares itself
for a pregnancy. If there is no pregnancy, the
corpus luteum starts to shrink and the level of
progesterone falls. The lining begins to break
down and, by day 27, the levels of oestrogen
and progesterone in the bloodstream are again
very low.

Day 28
Menstruation begins and so does a new cycle.

When Do You Ovulate?

Ovulation (the release of an egg) usually occurs
somewhere between 12 and 16 days before
your next period begins. Some women can

tell when they ovulate because they get a pain in their lower abdomen. Another sign that ovulation is about to occur is when the mucous from your cervix (the neck of the uterus) becomes thinner and more watery. You can feel this by inserting a finger into your vagina; the mucous will feel slippery and stretchy and look a bit like the white of an uncooked egg. Your temperature will also rise very slightly with ovulation and stay up until your next period.

What is PMS?

Premenstrual Syndrome (PMS), sometimes also called PMT (Premenstrual Tension), is the name given to the collection of symptoms that some women complain of with their periods. PMS is a very common problem for women of all ages. There has been little research into the causes of PMS, and many doctors don't know much about it and don't take it very seriously. No one really knows why some women suffer from PMS and others don't.

Common symptoms of PMS include:

- Swelling of abdomen, feet, ankles, breasts
- Headaches
- Weight gain
- Muscular or joint pain
- Abdominal pain – that dull ache or 'heavy' feeling
- Dizziness, tiredness

- Poor sleep
- Bowel problems
- Mood swings
- Anxiety and/or depression
- Food cravings.

What Can You Do about PMS?

Some women find that their symptoms are worse around the time of menopause. If you are having problems, there are many things you can try:

- Reduce your intake of salt, sugar, fats, caffeine
- Increase your intake of whole grain cereals, green leafy vegetables, water
- Take Vitamin B6 (pyrodoxine) up to 100 mg daily
- Take Vitamin B1, 50 mg daily (for sore breasts)
- Ask a naturopath about helpful minerals and herbs
- Ask your doctor about drugs available for specific symptoms
- Get plenty of exercise.

UNDERSTANDING YOUR SEXUAL ORGANS

It's really not surprising that so many women haven't got a clue about what they've got 'down there'. It's all so much easier for a man; his 'equipment' is always there for him to see whenever he goes to the toilet, not something that's hidden away, as it is for a woman.

As a little girl you were told by your anxious mother to 'wipe yourself clean, from front to back'. You were probably not encouraged to get a mirror and have a really good look at yourself. Have you ever seen your own clitoris or cervix?

The next time you have a smear, ask for a mirror so you can have a look. There's a treat in store for you!

Did you know that the largest and most important sexual organ that we have is . . . the brain! It is responsible for our fantasies, our memories, our imagination and our anticipation. On the negative side, it is also responsible for our hang-ups about sex, our sexual organs and our bodies. We often compare ourselves to the fantasy women and men created by the media and definitely find ourselves lacking! Men worry that their penises are not big enough and women worry that their breasts are too small or too large, or that they have cellulite on their thighs. No one ever talks much about body secretions and sexual odours on TV and, as we grow older, no one talks about the subtle changes in our bodies with ageing.

It's important to know what some of these changes are and why they happen. Your genitals, breasts, bladder, skin, hair and pelvic floor muscles are all dependent on oestrogen to keep them in tip-top condition.

CHANGES TO EXPECT

At menopause, with lowered levels of oestrogen, you may notice the following changes:

On the Outside

Vulva: This is the name given to your external sexual organs (the ones you can see), including the labia or lips, the clitoris, the pad of fat on top of your pubic bone and the pubic hair.

As you grow older, you may notice you have less pubic hair, less fatty tissue and that you feel 'drier' between your labia. You may even feel itchy or sore.

On the Inside

Uterus (womb): This will shrink in size. Prolapse can also occur at this time. This is when the uterus drops down into the vagina because the muscles which usually support it are weakened. The muscle tone in the pelvic area is affected by childbirth and menopause. You should do regular pelvic floor exercises to prevent this happening (see Chapter 5). Two other kinds of prolapses are when the bladder drops into the vagina (cystocele) and when the rectum drops into the vagina (rectocele).

Ovaries: These will start to shrink in size after a woman reaches the age of about 30. They also become less responsive to the pituitary hormones.

Vagina: The lining inside the vagina becomes thinner and the vagina shrinks in size. It doesn't expand as easily as it did before because there is less blood flow in the lining of the vaginal wall. Lubrication, which occurs when you become sexually aroused and feel 'wet' in the vagina, will take longer than before. The vagina becomes less acidic and you may be more likely to suffer from vaginal infections, such as thrush (candida).

Other Changes to Your Body

Bladder: Changes also occur in the neck of the bladder. The tissues become thinner and infections are more common. You may suffer from an 'irritable bladder', giving you the urge to urinate more frequently. You may also develop 'stress incontinence' when you cough, sneeze, laugh or play tennis. This can be due to weak pelvic floor muscles as well as to the weakened muscle tone of the bladder itself.

Breasts: As you grow older, there is a loss of both the elastic and gland tissue in the breasts. After menopause, some women's breasts become smaller while in other women they become larger, with increased fatty tissue. Your breasts will become less firm because there are fewer collagen fibres to support the tissue and skin.

Skin: Your skin is exposed to all sorts of harmful elements in the environment. Most people are aware of the damaging effects of the sun, but other factors, such as air pollution, diet, alcohol and smoking can also affect your skin. After the age of about 30, the number of collagen fibres decreases and there is also less water in the skin cells. This results in drier and thinner skin, the appearance of wrinkles, and sagging under the chin and on the upper arms and legs.

By the way, expensive moisturisers will not prevent this process, despite all the advertising claims. A simple, inexpensive moisturiser which contains sorbolene will help your dry skin. Taking oestrogen will help to reduce the loss of collagen and increase the water content of the cells. However, neither of these remedies will reverse the ageing process.

Itchy skin: 'Am I going crazy?' some women ask. 'My skin feels as though ants are crawling under it.' This can be a most frightening experience. No one really knows what the cause of this so-called 'formication' is, but it seems to be related to changing hormone and chemical levels in the bloodstream at menopause.

Hair: Some women notice changes in their hair after menopause. The tissue surrounding the hair follicles is mostly made up of collagen. When the amount of collagen decreases, it can cause some hair loss. You may also notice pubic and underarm hair loss, and an increase in hair on the face, arms and legs. These changes are due to lower oestrogen levels and increased androgen (male hormone) levels. Greying hair is often a different texture and can be coarse and dry. Some women notice that their hair may be more oily than before.

Weight gain or 'middle-aged spread': You may put on extra weight around the time of menopause and notice changes in your body shape, such as thickening of the waistline and fat on your upper arms or back. As you grow older your metabolism slows down and you don't burn up as many kilojoules as before. If you continue to eat the same amount of food and don't increase your level of physical activity, then you will gain weight.

After menopause, women have higher levels of the androgens (male hormones) which promote the deposit of fat, particularly around the abdomen. The body can easily convert this fat to oestrogen when it is needed. Perhaps the extra fat is nature's way of storing up oestrogen reserves. Weight gain can also be due to the increase in fatty tissue which can retain fluid.

Aches and pains: In some women, when their hormone levels fall, the ligaments which hold the bones together lose their elasticity and the muscles become less firm. This can cause muscle and joint aches and pains, particularly in the knees, ankles, shoulders and back. Arthritis can also become a problem for some women with swelling of the joints, particularly in the fingers and hands.

Palpitations: Palpitations are a fluttering sensation in your heart that may last for a few seconds or minutes. They may be related to menopause but can also be caused by caffeine, nicotine, anxiety or fear. If you have them frequently, see your doctor because they can also be a symptom of heart disease.

Sleep disturbances: Insomnia, or poor sleep, can be caused by hot flushes and sweating at night. Some doctors believe that lower levels of oestrogen affect the sleep centre in the brain. Poor sleep can also be due to other causes, such as anxiety or depression, drinking coffee or tea late at night, lack of exercise, or going to bed on a full stomach. And, finally, of course:

Those 'Famous' Hot Flushes

These are the most common symptoms of menopause and are often associated with other symptoms, such as:

- Sweating – particularly in bed at night
- Palpitations
- Sleep disturbances
- Dizziness
- Numbness and tingling in the legs.

Hot flushes are such a widespread and troubling symptom of menopause that they deserve special attention. A hot flush is a sudden sensation of intense heat which may be accompanied by perspiration and reddening of the skin. This can happen over the entire body, but the face, neck and upper body are the most common places. It can last from a few seconds to several minutes and occasionally even longer.

The number of hot flushes that women experience can vary from a few each month to as many as 40 or 50 a day. They are usually more common at night, particularly in bed. Sweating may also be a problem and you may need to change your sheets and nightwear.

Q. *How long will I have them?*
A. This varies with each individual. They may start years before you have your last period and continue for a few years afterwards. A small number of women go on having them for many years after the menopause, a few even until they are 60 or 70!

Q. *What causes them?*
A. No one knows exactly. They are believed to be related to changing levels of hormones and chemicals in the bloodstream. Hot flushes can be triggered by any change in your environment – including emotional changes (such as anxiety or excitement) and physical changes (such as temperature, hot spicy foods, caffeine or alcohol).

Chapter 3
Not Seeing Red but Feeling Blue

There are particular times in people's lives that are especially significant, but it's the weight the individual gives them that makes them important. One landmark may be of consequence to one individual and not to another.

(William H. Masters, M.D.)

This statement holds true for menopause and mid-life. The important question to ask yourself is:

'WHAT DOES MENOPAUSE MEAN TO ME?'

Your answer will depend on where you are and what's happening in your life at the moment, what your past experiences have been and what sort of picture you have of the future. Perhaps you see mid-life as a sign of getting old or you may see it as an exciting new phase of your life – a time when you are free to develop your own interests. It may be that it doesn't mean very much to you at all.

Your reaction to menopause may be influenced by other people's expectations of you, particularly of those who are close to you. The stereotypical picture of a woman at menopause is often a very negative one.

It's interesting to look at other cultures where menopause is regarded in a more positive way than in our own youth-oriented one. In these cultures, women often look forward to menopause as a time when they may then be given new privileges and freedom.

Menopause is still not widely discussed. When it is mentioned, for example in the media, it is often presented as a medical condition that needs to be treated like an illness.

OTHER CHANGES ARE HAPPENING, TOO

It is important to remember that menopause is only one event in mid-life. There are many changes and new situations to face at this time, and change can be very challenging. Our life cycle is all about changes and choices. We are constantly meeting new challenges and new situations and are required to make all sorts of decisions. In childhood and adolescence we grow and develop very rapidly. Much of our learning about ourselves is influenced by those around us, in particular by our parents and friends.

As young adults we are faced with many decisions – choosing a career, finding a partner, whether to have children and where to live. In mid-life, we may have ageing parents to take care of. We may have to cope with the demands of adolescent children, illness in the family or the loss of those we love.

How we adjust to these changes will vary with each individual. Some of us will adjust easily to changing situations, while others may have more difficulty in coping.

WHAT'S GOING ON AT HOME?

Menopause occurs at a time when there may be many stressful events in your life. Having to cope with these and the symptoms of menopause at the same time may be overwhelming for some women. It seems that menopause, with its effects on hormonal balance and body metabolism, may make you more vulnerable in stressful situations and lower your ability to cope with them.

Stress can affect every hormone level in your body. Acute stress, occurring as a sudden reaction to a stressful situation, raises levels of certain hormones. Chronic stress, present for a long period of time, can lower hormone levels, particularly sex hormones. Common examples of this stress-related effect are irregular periods and heavy bleeding in women with emotional distress and in men, impotence (the inability to have an erection of the penis). There seem to be three common pictures:

- Some women are more sensitive to hormonal changes at menopause. These women will suffer symptoms even though everything is OK in their life at that time.
- Some women have very stressful life events at the time of menopause which may increase their symptoms.
- Some women can cope with both the hormonal changes and the stressful life events much better than others.

Carrying the load: Your family expects you to be a constant source of emotional support, always there no matter what other problems you may have, and always ready to listen.

Often there is no one to give you the same support when you need it. These days it is quite common for a woman to have the responsibility for not only the emotional support of her family but the financial one as well. It takes an enormous amount of energy to balance all these demands and still leave some extra time for yourself.

A man about the house: Women at mid-life often become more radical and assertive; men, on the other hand, may become more conservative and less assertive. If you have a male partner, he may become increasingly dependent on you for emotional support, particularly when he retires from work.

'I married him for better or for worse, but not for lunch!' – this is often the main complaint from women who suddenly find their man around the house all day. He may want a bit of nurturing and resents it when you go out and leave him. 'Helpful' suggestions about how to streamline the household chores, when you have been managing quite well for the last 20 or 30 years, are also a bit hard to take!

Ageing parents: At this time, you may have ageing parents who are becoming more frail and less independent. You may also have the responsibility for parents-in-law. Just as you have launched your children into the world as young adults, your own parents are becoming more childlike and demanding your attention.

Poor health and chronic illness: You or your partner may experience the beginning of a chronic illness, such as arthritis, diabetes, high blood pressure or cancer. Some of your friends may also become ill or develop diseases. You may become anxious and worried, not only about them, but about your own health as well.

EMPTY NEST . . .

Mid-life usually coincides with the adolescence of your children. It can be a turbulent time for everyone when the children begin to loosen their ties and become independent. When children leave home, for whatever reason, it is a time of adjustment for them and for you.

The so-called 'empty nest syndrome' is the term given to the feelings of loss that some women experience when their children leave home. If you have concentrated all your energies on your children, you may feel that your whole reason for living has suddenly gone. This is more likely to occur if you have few outside interests, don't work outside the home, perhaps live alone or if your relationship with your partner is not a happy one.

If this description fits you, it is important that you think about what else you can do with your life, beyond your role as a mother. Now is the time to take up something that interests you. It doesn't matter whether it is a job, a hobby, sport or study. The important thing is to find something that will enable you to express yourself in a way that raises your self-esteem. Feeling good about yourself as a person, not just as Mum, will help you cope with the 'empty nest'.

. . . OR PATTER OF BIG FEET

One of the big changes in society today is that children are not leaving home or are leaving home much later than in the past. Finding they are unable to support themselves financially, they may leave home and then return – not once, but several times!

Just as you are beginning to enjoy your new

freedom and have redecorated their room, your child is back. This can put an enormous strain on you, your partner and other members of the family as well.

Having tasted freedom, your newly arrived young adult may not take too kindly to you imposing house rules as you did before. Be strong – remember, if they want to enjoy the benefits, they have to be prepared for a bit of give as well as take.

STRESS, LOSS AND COPING

Q. *What is stress?*
A. People talk a lot about stress these days. Sometimes the word is used to mean anxiety, tension or stress. Stress is actually the reaction of our bodies to a situation that makes us feel anxious, frightened or angry. The important thing about stress is not the situation that triggers it, but how each individual sees the situation and reacts to it. What causes you to be stressed may not affect someone else in the same way.

Positive and Negative Stress

A certain amount of stress is necessary to motivate us and keep us involved in daily living. Even pleasant things, like going on a holiday, moving into a new house or having friends for dinner, can be stressful.

Negative stress occurs when a situation affects us, causing both physical and emotional problems. When you confront a stressful situation, your body releases a hormone called adrenalin, which prepares you to deal with the situation. It is sometimes called the flight or fight response. In other words, your body prepares you for running from the situation or for defending yourself in some way.

To do either of these things you will need more oxygen, so you start to breathe more quickly. Other changes include: faster heart beat, raised blood pressure, sweating, and body hair standing on end (goose bumps on the skin).

The cause of your stress is called a stressor. Someone with many stressors in their life can experience chronic stress. Eventually, this can lead to exhaustion.

Q. *What can I do about stress?*
A. There are many ways of handling stress. Find one that works for you. Some of the ways include:

- If possible, avoid situations that are stressful
- Don't try to do everything at once
- Talk to someone about your feelings
- Don't worry too much about the past or the future
- Learn to relax
- Get plenty of sleep
- Get plenty of exercise.

LIFE IS FULL OF LOSSES

At some time, we will all experience the loss of separation, either through death or through the breakdown of relationships. Other losses, such as the loss of a job, financial losses or even loss through missed opportunities, are a part of life.

Some women will also experience the loss of some part of their body, such as the breast or the womb, as a result of a life-threatening illness or disease. How an individual reacts to a loss will depend, to a large extent, on how that person views that loss and what it means to them. The effects of loss and grief can be severe. They can even cause a lowering of our immune system to such an extent that we can become more liable to illness.

Each of us has different ways of coping with loss and some of us can cope much better than others. Resolving grief from any loss is a long process.

You will need support from those around you and it may take a long time for you to accept the loss. You may need to seek professional help to enable you to work through your grief and resolve it in a healthy way.

LEARNING HOW TO COPE

It's a fact that coping gives you a feeling of control. Some of us are born with the ability to cope with life's challenges better than others.

If you are not one of these fortunate people, you can still learn new skills to help you get through. When you learn to cope with difficult challenges, you will be better able to take charge of your life.

You have three options for dealing with difficult situations:

- You can let it all wash over you, like the waves, but you risk being tossed about all over the place.
- You can bury your head in the sand and pretend nothing's wrong at all.
- You can start to work out some new ways of dealing with the problem.

This last way of dealing with difficult situations begins with seeing things as they really are. It may mean taking a good, long look at yourself, which in itself can be difficult. It also means making decisions and sticking to them, which may lead to conflict with those around you, especially if it involves them in change of some kind.

DEPRESSION – 'IS IT ALL IN MY HEAD?'

Everyone feels down or miserable once in a while. Sometimes, everything seems to be going wrong. In this situation, we often blame ourselves and have very negative thoughts. For example:

'Where did I go wrong?'
You may feel guilty that your children haven't achieved what you had hoped they would or you just can't seem to relate to them at all. You blame yourself.

'What could I have done differently?'
Your own career or your partner's may not have been as successful as you had anticipated. Your marriage or your relationship may have been a failure. You feel bitter and sad.

'Why do I feel so angry?'
You resent the time you have to spend caring for your elderly parents or parents-in-law. You feel guilty.

'What's there to look forward to?'
Everything looks so grey and bleak. Nothing seems as bright any more, even the colours of the flowers, the sky and the trees all look dull. You feel miserable.

There is a big difference between feeling miserable, angry, anxious or guilty, now and then, and having a depressive illness.

Mood changes are very common at menopause, and it's hard to know whether this is due to changing hormone levels or to other factors operating in your life at this time. Depression can sometimes occur as a reaction to a crisis, such as divorce, separation or the death of someone you love.

Sometimes, a crisis that occurs in later life can trigger a severe depression because of an earlier loss that you may have experienced, such as the death of a parent when you were a child. Some people seem to be more prone to depression than others. Many doctors believe that depression is caused by biochemical changes in the brain.

Q. *What are the symptoms of depression?*
A. You may be in need of help if the following apply to you:

- Feeling tired all the time with no energy
- Feeling sad and crying a lot
- Disturbed sleep, waking up and unable to go back to sleep
- Disturbed appetite, eating very little or far too much
- Dry mouth
- Increase in smoking or drinking alcohol
- Weight loss
- Difficulty making minor decisions
- Feelings of guilt and self-blame
- Loss of interest in sex
- Aches and pains
- Thoughts of suicide.

Q. *What can I do about it?*
A. It's important to talk to someone about how you are feeling. Your family and friends will probably notice that you are sad and not your usual self, but not understand why. You may not fully understand why you are depressed either. Talking things over with an understanding person who is close to you may be helpful.

You may prefer to seek professional help,

rather than have your friends and family know just how depressed you really are. Depressive illness still has a certain stigma attached to it, as though it is some sort of weakness, which of course it's not.

Professional help is available, but it might take a few tries until you find the person who is right for you. You could choose a trained counsellor, such as a psychologist, a family therapist or a psychiatrist. If you need medication, you will need to be in the care of a doctor.

TRANQUILLISERS AND SEDATIVES

These medications should only be used as a temporary support. Unfortunately, many women are prescribed them for long periods of time and can become dependent, as some of them are addictive.

During times of severe stress, you may be unable to sleep or to relax. Eventually, you will be worn out and even less able to cope with your problems. Sedatives, sleeping pills and tranquillisers can be very useful during these times. They will help you to get proper rest at night so you will have more energy to cope with the problems during the day. They won't make the problems disappear.

Q. *Will a stiff drink help?*
A. One, or even two, drinks a day may have some beneficial effects. Alcohol can help you to relax and may even reduce your risk of certain

types of heart disease. Unfortunately, some women don't stop with just one or two drinks and may increase their drinking to help them cope. The effects of this excessive intake, especially if combined with tranquillisers, can be disastrous. If you think that you have a drinking problem, seek professional help.

ANTIDEPRESSANTS

These are sometimes prescribed by doctors for depressive illness and should always be taken under strict medical supervision. They are not addictive and will take about three weeks to have any effect on your depression. There may be some side effects when you take these drugs, such as a dry mouth. You should also be careful with alcohol; alcohol and antidepressants do not mix very well at all. When your doctor feels that you no longer need medication, you should taper off the dose slowly and not suddenly stop taking them.

IS MENOPAUSE TO BLAME?

Menopause will not cause a depressive illness; in fact depression is more common in women in their late thirties. There is a tendency for depressive illness to recur. If you recognise the symptoms and begin to feel as you did before, see your doctor immediately. There is nothing to be ashamed about in seeking help for a depressive illness.

Chapter 4
Sexuality:
A Change for the Better?

We are all sexual beings from the moment we are born until the moment we die. Sexuality is not just about sex, it is an integral part of our personality, unique to each one of us and constantly changing. It is about who we are, how we see ourselves and how we express ourselves in our relationships.

At menopause, you might find it hard to feel really good about yourself, for many reasons. You might believe that you are no longer sexually attractive or that you will no longer feel like having sex. A relationship may have ended or may no longer be happy.

Any of these things, coupled with the unpleasant physical symptoms that you may be experiencing, can make you lose confidence in yourself.

Many people reach adulthood with much anxiety about their own sexuality, resulting from poor childhood experiences, misinformation or no information at all. Older women may have added anxieties about their desirability, because of the way that our society tends to devalue them.

GOOD SEX BEGINS IN THE KITCHEN

Many women complain that the only time their partner wants to communicate with them is in bed by having sex. It is often said that women need to feel close to have sex and that men need to have sex to feel close. Are we really that different or is that what we have been conditioned to believe?

People have sex for all kinds of reasons – to release tension, to express love, to get closer to someone, to get to sleep, because they think they should and for other, more sinister reasons, such as exerting power and control over a partner.

Sex is not always enjoyable for both partners, especially when it is without any true feelings of tenderness and concern for the other person. Some women say that they often feel used during sex, if there is no real communication at any other time.

Good sex does not mean penis in vagina sex only. Sexual expression can take many different forms. Sometimes, it may just be touching, stroking, cuddling, kissing, massaging or having a bath together. Often, the best sex happens spontaneously, when neither partner feels pressured to have intercourse.

THERE IS NO SUCH THING AS 'NORMAL' SEX

Any form of sexual expression between two people that is enjoyable for both of them is good. It really does not matter what you do, how you do it, where you do it, how often or how little you do it. What does matter is that you both feel good about it.

No one should be pressured to have sex or to do something they find unpleasant or painful.

Men and women often have very negative attitudes towards sex as a result of childhood experiences, parental or religious influences and past sexual experiences. Some women, and men too, have been victims of sexual assault which can have lasting effects on their future relationships.

Older women may believe that they should not be having sexual feelings after menopause at all which, of course, is not true. Some women may have never had strong sexual feelings, others may find their sexual feelings are stronger than ever before.

Sexual feelings do not exist in a vacuum. What is going on in your life will determine, to a large extent, how you feel about sex. The quality of the relationship with your partner will affect the quality of your sexual experience.

Where there is tension, anger, tiredness, anxiety or mistrust, the level of sexual satisfaction will be extremely low. Boredom is a big turn-off. If you have had sex every Saturday night in the same way for 25 years with no variation, you could hardly be expected to enjoy it very much.

You will face many things in mid-life which can affect your sexuality. These may include:

- Society's negative attitudes to older women
- How you see yourself; there may be a belief that you are no longer sexually attractive because you are no longer young
- Poor relationship with your partner
- Loss of your partner
- A new partner
- Illness, surgery, loss
- Other stressful life events.

SEX WITHOUT A PARTNER

Many women are alone at mid-life. You may have never been in a long-term sexual relationship or, in fact, in any relationship. That does not mean that you are asexual or have no sexual feelings.

For many people, masturbation still has a negative image as a result of countless years of myths and taboos. Masturbation is a completely natural form of sexual expression. The body responds in exactly the same way through self-stimulation as it does with intercourse.

You should not feel guilty in any way about masturbation. In fact, both women and men continue to masturbate throughout their life,

with or without a sexual partner. It is not only
good for you, it is enjoyable!

'COMING OUT' AT MID-LIFE

Some women decide at mid-life to openly
acknowledge their sexual preference and, for
the first time, may begin a relationship with
someone of the same sex.

These feelings may have been suppressed all
their life while they married and had children.
The reaction from family and friends may be
one of disbelief and dismay. People are general-
ly more accepting of homosexuality today, but
it can still be a difficult time for all concerned. In
the future, with many more women outliving
men, we may see this 'coming out' occurring far
more frequently than in the past.

YOUR SEX DRIVE

Sexual desire, libido or what 'turns you on'
varies from woman to woman. For most women, a feeling of closeness, a touch and a little
bit of fantasy is all that is needed. It is also
important for you to feel good about yourself.

Lack of sexual desire is often associated with
underlying problems in relationships. It can also
be affected by such things as poor health,
medication, anxiety, depression, financial and
other worries, and tiredness.

There is no need to feel anxious if you don't feel much sexual desire: there are many good, long-lasting relationships that are not dependent on sexual intercourse to maintain them. It does not mean that there is something wrong with you if you don't feel like sex.

Some women say that they are less interested in sex after menopause, others say it is more enjoyable than ever. One sure way to improve your sex drive is to have an interested (and interesting) partner.

SEXUAL RESPONSE

Sexual response is as much to do with what is in our head as it is with what is in our vagina. Many doctors talk about menopause and a dry vagina as if that is all that matters. Fix up the dry vagina and bingo – instant sexual response! Women are not like cars – an oil and grease are not the only requirements for a smoothly running machine or a satisfactory sex life.

It is true that the decrease in hormone levels at menopause means that vaginal lubrication during sexual arousal may take longer – anything from one to five minutes. Often, changes in the vagina, such as thinner walls, shortening and narrowing, less acidity and an increased incidence of vaginal infections can combine to make sexual intercourse painful. However, not all women experience these changes.

Regular sexual activity, either through intercourse or masturbation, can improve lubrication and blood flow to the vaginal walls. Hormone replacement therapy will also have a beneficial effect on the vagina, improving the lubrication and thickening the vaginal walls. The use of a water-based lubricant can also relieve discomfort during intercourse. Pelvic floor exercises are important to strengthen muscle tone. (See Chapter 5.)

The clitoris, which is the most sensitive and important area for women during sexual response, is still alive and well after menopause. If the labia are dry and have lost a lot of their fatty tissue, then the clitoris is more exposed and too much friction can cause discomfort. Our skin sensitivity is still intact after menopause.

Other areas of our body, such as the breasts, thighs, back, neck, mouth and bottom, all continue to respond to touch as before. In fact, many women say that these areas become increasingly sensitive and responsive as they grow older.

Contractions of the uterus and vagina during orgasm may be fewer in number and may be less intense. This does seem to vary a lot. Some women say that their orgasms are better than ever. If you have large fibroids in your uterus, contractions during orgasm can sometimes cause pain.

MEN AT MID-LIFE

There is no such thing as male menopause. How could there be? Men do not menstruate. It's a catchy phrase, but it has no meaning.

However, men do experience some similar physical and emotional changes at mid-life. They share many of the same problems, such as ageing parents, adolescent children, ill-health, retirement and stressful life events.

Obvious physical changes in men are greying hair or loss of hair, wrinkles, weight-gain and loss of muscle tone. There is also a slight shrinkage of the testes, erections are less frequent and are not as hard as they once were. It may take longer to ejaculate and much longer to have another erection, after ejaculating.

Impotence (the inability to have or sustain an erection) can be very worrying for men. Many men believe that penetration (penis/vagina sex) is the only real way to have sex. Of course, this is simply not true.

If your partner becomes impotent, help him to feel less anxious and reassure him that there are other enjoyable ways to have sex. There could be an underlying medical problem which is the cause of his impotence, such as diabetes, side effects of medication or poor circulation. An enlarged prostate gland can cause pain during erection or ejaculation and bladder problems.

Men at mid-life can often become depressed. They may feel that they have not been successful in their career or that their children have not achieved as much as they had hoped. Some men look for a younger woman to restore their flagging self-esteem. As men approach mid-life, they sometimes become more conservative in their attitudes. This can cause problems, especially if their partner is moving in the opposite direction, wanting to pursue new interests.

Many men find it difficult to relate to their adolescent children. They may not have had the opportunity to be close to them, during their growing years, because of the demands of work. Now that they have more time, they find it hard to make contact and can't understand why their adolescent children don't really want to be involved with them.

Women often become more assertive as they get older and have more energy. Men, on the other hand, often become less assertive, wanting to be nurtured and taken care of. It may be necessary to make a lot of changes in your relationship and set some new ground rules, in order to be more accepting of each other.

PREGNANT – WHO ME?

From the age of 40 it is likely that you will not ovulate regularly each month as before. There will be some months when you will not ovulate at all. You will become less fertile after the age of 40, but this does not mean that you can't become pregnant. As long as you are having periods, there is a possibility of a pregnancy. You will need to continue contraception (birth control) until you are sure that you are no longer ovulating. This will mean that you will need to use contraception until you have not had a period for at least 12 months

Choose the method that suits you	
Contraceptive methods available include:	
Hormonal:	low dose combined pill (oestrogen & progestogen) progestogen-only pill post-coital pill (morning after pill) Depo Provera injection
Intrauterine Device (IUD) Barrier Methods:	condoms diaphragms, cervical caps
Periodic Abstinence	natural family planning
Coitus Interruptus	withdrawal
Spermicides	foams, creams, jellies, pessaries
Permanent Sterilisation	tubal ligation (for you) vasectomy (for him)

Q. *What method of contraception should I choose?*
A. Your ideal contraceptive will depend on

what you and your partner find acceptable, on your general health and menstrual cycle. There are many different types of contraceptives to choose from. One of the best places to find out about contraception is from the Family Planning Association (see Helpful Addresses page 101). Your doctor or gynaecologist can also give you advice about contraception.

There is no ideal contraceptive for any age group. Some contraceptives may not be suitable for you because of your age, state of health, if you smoke or because of other lifestyle factors.

STDs – NOT JUST A LONG DISTANCE PHONE CALL

There is always a risk of getting a sexually transmitted disease (STD) whenever people have sex. If neither you nor your partner have an STD and neither of you have sex with anyone else outside your relationship, then you do not need to worry.

An older woman may be more at risk of certain infections, such as HIV/AIDS, because her vagina may be drier, with thinner walls, and she may have slight tearing of the vagina during intercourse.

Unfortunately many people are unaware that their partner has been having sex with someone else, until they become infected with an STD themselves. If you are concerned that this may be a possibility, then you need to think about safe sex practices.

Some methods of contraception, such as condoms (and to a lesser extent, diaphragms), will protect you against many STDs. Another way to have safer sex is to masturbate each other instead of having penetration. Oral sex can also put you at risk of getting some STDs if your partner has an infection.

If you have a new partner or suspect your partner may be at risk of getting an STD, discuss your worries about infection and use condoms until your partner has a checkup. You should also have a checkup, if you think you are at risk of getting an STD. If one of you does have an infection, then you will both have to be treated at the same time.

Q. *How do I tell if I have an STD or vaginal infection?*
A. If you have any unusual discharge from your vagina, pain on intercourse, blisters or sores on your vulval area, then you may have an infection. There are some STDs, occurring in women, that have no symptoms at all. If you feel unwell or have any pelvic pain, you should see a doctor. Regular cervical smears are also very important. (See Chapter 8.)

Chapter 5
Taking Care of You

Remember the old saying 'Prevention is better than cure'? The medical profession has taken a long time to move away from its emphasis on the treatment of disease to the new preventive health focus that is so popular today. Unfortunately, there are still some doctors who are reluctant to let go of the old model. These doctors view menopause, a natural event in a woman's life, as a disease that needs to be treated and managed.

Drug companies and some doctors, emphasising the long-term effects of lack of oestrogen, would have us believe that every woman over the age of 50 should receive treatment for the rest of her life. There <u>are</u> alternatives to taking synthetic drugs that change a woman's hormonal balance.

Health means more than just being disease-free. It also means feeling good about yourself, about the world you live in and about the degree of control you have over your own life.

Menopause is a time to look carefully at your lifestyle and how it might affect your health. It may be that you will need to make a few changes in order to feel healthier. If you eat well, get some regular exercise, learn some ways to reduce stress and be kinder to yourself, not only will you start to feel better, but you will look better as well. The symptoms that you thought were due to menopause or you had been told were 'to be expected at your age' may also disappear.

YOU ARE WHAT YOU EAT

What we choose to eat and drink is often influenced by our mood and habits. Most women reach menopause having been brainwashed into believing that they are overweight. For many women, life has been a constant round of diets of some kind or another.

At menopause, the appearance of extra weight around the waistline or a bit of extra flab under the arms, chin or thighs is enough to send many women into emotional decline. The media propaganda about being slim, beautiful and young has been well and truly learned by most women. We have been bombarded by images of anorexic-looking models, many of whom are probably not much older than 14 or 15. To be fat, 40 or 50 years old and no longer fertile is seen as being on the scrap-heap.

Being a <u>little</u> overweight at mid-life is probably not such a bad thing. Your body is able to convert some of your fat into oestrogen when needed, helping to diminish the effects of lowered hormone levels.

On the other hand, being a <u>lot</u> overweight is a definite health risk. If you are overweight, you are more likely to develop diabetes, diseases of the heart and circulation, gall-bladder disorders and joint problems. Your heart, lungs and digestive system have to work a lot harder if you are overweight. Think of the added strain on your back and legs as well.

Most women notice an increase in weight at this stage of life. Often there is a redistribution of weight as well. You may notice a thickening around your waist, shoulders or back. Your body metabolism slows down as you grow older and you might exercise less. If you continue to eat the same amount of food as before, then you will put on weight. If your weight is OK and you exercise regularly, you probably don't need to worry too much about the kilojoules, but you should reduce the amount that you eat.

The best diet for menopause and mid-life is one that is high in whole grains, vegetables, fruit and calcium-rich foods. You should try and eat foods that will give you as many nutrients as possible for the number of kilojoules taken in.

Eating Well for Menopause and Mid-Life

Drink plenty of water

Drinking 6 to 8 glasses of water a day is essential for good health. Water facilitates all the chemical reactions in your body. It helps carbohydrates, proteins and fats release energy, as well as speeding up the movement of nutrients.

Eat most of these foods

Bread (wholemeal and wholegrain)
Pasta, rice and cereal foods
These contain starch for energy and protein for building muscle and body tissues. They are also a major source of thiamin (vitamin B1) and an important source of the minerals, zinc and iron. Bread and cereals also contain dietary fibre which is important for a healthy bowel.

Vegetables, dried peas, beans,
lentils and fruit
These provide some starch, low concentrations of sugar, vitamins, minerals and dietary fibre. Vegetables and fruit are high in vitamin C and beta-carotene which the body can turn into vitamin A. The dietary fibre in these foods helps to lower blood cholesterol levels.

Eat moderate amounts of these foods

Lean meat, poultry without the skin, and fish, nuts, eggs, milk, cheese and yoghurt
These foods are rich in protein, used to build and repair muscle, blood and other body tissues. Important vitamins in milk, meat, chicken, fish and eggs are riboflavin, niacin and thiamin (vitamin BI) and vitamin BI2. Minerals found in meat are zinc and iron. Milk, cheese and yoghurt also contain calcium. These foods can also contain fat, so choose low fat milks, cheese and yoghurt wherever possible.

Eat small amounts of these foods

Butter, table margarine, oil
These foods are high in fats and can raise blood cholesterol levels.

Sugar
This is a carbohydrate which provides energy, but no vitamins, minerals, fibre or protein.

Salt
Salt, or sodium chloride, is found in many foods. We probably get much more salt than we need, so don't add any to food. Excess salt can increase fluid retention and may raise blood pressure.   (cont.)

Caffeine

This is a stimulant found in coffee, tea, chocolate and cola soft drinks. It can be addictive and in high doses can cause irritability, tension, increased and irregular heart beats, raised blood pressure, diarrhoea, erratic blood sugar levels and increased urinary frequency. Caffeine can also increase the frequency of hot flushes, benign breast lumps, breast pain and the loss of calcium and other essential vitamins and minerals. If you have a large amount of caffeine each day, you should try to reduce the amount slowly. If you stop suddenly, you can suffer from withdrawal symptoms, such as headaches and irritability.

VITAMINS AND MINERALS

Vitamins are naturally occurring chemical substances that are vital to life. Minerals are minute quantities of certain elements that are needed for cell function and to enable vitamin activity to take place.

Some of the problems women have at menopause may be related to low levels of some vitamins and minerals. Increasing your intake, either by natural means or by taking supplements, may help to relieve some of your symptoms. Taking vitamin and mineral supplements can be an expensive business. If you take too many, your body will excrete some, but some can be stored in the body and become toxic (e.g., vitamin A).

During periods of physical and emotional stress, your body uses up more of these nutrients than normal. The best way to ensure that your body has enough vitamins and minerals is to eat a balanced diet, reduce your intake of caffeine, alcohol and salt, drink plenty of water and don't smoke.

Should I Take Supplements?

If you are going to take supplements, consult your doctor or a naturopath who is a specialist in this area. Some supplements can cause an allergic reaction or gastric upsets.

Vitamin B Complex and Vitamin C: These help the body to cope with physical and emotional stress. Vitamin C is an antioxidant that helps to protect you against free radicals which can damage your cells. Skin cells are particularly vulnerable, resulting in ageing changes, such as thinning of the skin and wrinkles. Vitamin C also helps to fight infections and allergic reactions.

Vitamin E: Natural vitamin E supplements can help control hot flushes, but you may need to take them for weeks or months before they have any effect. They retard cell ageing, reduce tiredness and help to keep your veins healthy.

Vitamin D: This helps the body to absorb

calcium. It is activated in the body by sunlight. Too much of this vitamin can be toxic.

Vitamin K: This is important in forming substances that enable your blood to clot properly.

Vitamin A: This can also be toxic, if you take too much, as it is stored in the body. It is necessary for the healthy function of the skin, and lining of the stomach and lungs.

Beta-carotene: This is converted into vitamin A in the liver. It is an antioxidant and is helpful in preventing drying of mucous membranes (linings) in the body. If you take too much, your skin can turn a yellow or bronze colour.

Calcium: This mineral is important at menopause, particularly if you choose not to take oestrogen replacement treatment. Calcium is discussed in detail in Chapter 6.

Other Supplements

Evening Primrose Oil: This is rich in unsaturated fatty acids, mainly linoleic and gamma linoleic acids (GLA). GLA deficiency may affect PMS, arthritic conditions, your moods, and the condition of your skin, hair and nails. It may also help control hot flushes, dry vagina and itching eyes.

Max EPA: EPA (eicosapentaenoic acid) is found in cod liver oil. It helps control blood clotting and lowers cholesterol and triglyceride levels.

BEST OF ALL – TRY EXERCISE

As you grow older, exercise is one of the most important things that you can do. Not only will you feel better, you'll look better too. The benefits of regular exercise are:

- You will maintain your ideal weight
- You will be less likely to develop osteoporosis (weakening of your bones)
- You will not feel stiff in your joints or have as many aches and pains (unless you overdo the exercise)
- You will have more energy and reduce your level of stress
- You will be reducing your risk of heart disease
- You will sleep better
- You will improve your bowel function (no more constipation).

Q. *What kind of exercise should I do?*
A. If you start to exercise after many years of little or no physical activity – start slowly! If you have any medical problems, check with your doctor before you begin. There are many activities that provide healthy and enjoyable exercise. Many of these will also have the added benefit of enabling you to meet new people. Tennis, golf, walking and dancing are all good weight-control exercises that help to keep bones healthy and strong. They will also im-

prove your heart, circulation and lungs. Aerobic exercises to music or a session at a gym are also beneficial. Cycling and swimming are good exercise, but are not weight-bearing, so you would need to walk for at least 30 minutes, three times a week, as well. Jogging on a hard surface can cause back, knee and ankle problems. Brisk walking is just as good and much kinder to your joints.

Stretching exercises, such as yoga and Tai Chi, help your joints and improve your muscle tone, as well as reducing stress.

Pelvic Floor Exercises

Your pelvic floor muscles stretch from your pubic bone across to the bottom of your tail bone like a tight hammock. They hold your bladder, uterus and bowel in place. These muscles are often weakened due to childbirth, injury, lack of exercise and menopause. If the muscles start to sag, you may be more likely to have a prolapse of your uterus. You may also have problems with your bladder, such as loss of control and leaking of urine. Doing pelvic floor exercises will improve your bladder control and vaginal response during sex.

Q. *How can I tell if the muscles are weak?*
A. There are a couple of simple tests you can do yourself:

- Insert two fingers gently into your vagina when you are propped up in a half-sitting position in bed. If your vagina is dry, use some water-based lubricant or saliva on your fingers. Close your eyes and concentrate. Pull up your muscles as though you were trying to stop yourself passing wind. How many times can you pull up and hold for 2 seconds? Rest for 4 seconds between each contraction.

- Sit on the toilet with your knees wide apart and try to stop the flow of urine. You should be able to stop the flow completely. Only try this once a day.

- First count how many contractions you can manage without getting tired. Then aim to increase the number gradually and continue to do the exercises several times a day. You can do them under the shower, on the toilet, on the phone, in your car or anywhere at all. No one will know what you're up to!

If you are unable to manage the exercises and need a bit of help, see a physiotherapist who is experienced in treating pelvic floor muscles.

Q. *How long do I have to do them?*
A. Every day for the rest of your life!

WHAT ABOUT ALTERNATIVE THERAPIES?

Many women seek help for their menopause problems from alternative forms of treatment to those offered by traditional medicine. Some of these may be beneficial, others may prove to be harmful. If you do choose to try one of these therapies, make sure that the person you see is qualified and experienced in their field.

Herbal Remedies: Medicinal extracts or herbal teas can be used to treat a number of symptoms that are due to hormonal changes at menopause. Herbal remedies are usually given in combination with advice about nutrition. It is important to see a qualified herbalist before taking any herbal remedies.

Naturopathy: A naturopath believes in the ability of the body to heal itself. Attention is given to the diet and the reduction of bad habits, which may be affecting the natural harmony of the body. Some naturopaths also recommend natural dietary supplements.

Acupuncture: The fundamental principle of acupuncture is also based on the body's ability to heal itself. There are pathways of energy throughout the body which, if disturbed in some way, can alter the body's natural balance. An acupuncturist uses needles placed at certain focal points to restore the normal flow of energy.

Homeopathy: Homeopathic remedies are also concerned with body harmony. They are given to produce similar symptoms to those that are occurring in the body, encourage the body to restore itself to natural harmony and overcome the disease process.

Reflexology: Reflexologists believe that there is a life force which flows along ten channels in the body, beginning in the toes. Pressure, applied to the feet at different locations, stimulates a reflex which affects particular organs.

Hypnotherapy: A hypnotherapist can help to reduce stress, and anxiety, assist with overcoming dependence on alcohol and cigarettes, and help you to manage physical symptoms that do not appear to have a cause.

Massage: A massage can be one of the biggest treats you can give yourself. It relaxes you, relieves tension and helps all your aches and pains. It also stimulates your circulation.

VAGINAL VITALITY

Keeping your vagina healthy at menopause is a must. Normally, your vagina is quite capable of looking after itself, but as you get older and have lowered levels of circulating oestrogen, you may need to take more care.

The vagina depends on oestrogen to keep it in tip-top condition. Anything that disturbs the normal acid/alkaline balance or the normal organisms that live in the vagina can cause problems. Stress, illness, diet, taking antibiotics or other drugs, can all affect this normal balance.

Q. *What's healthy?*
A. A normal vaginal secretion is whitish, with its own distinct smell. It dries to a yellowish colour on your underpants. In women who are still having periods, it is lighter and heavier at different times of the month.

Q. *What's unhealthy?*
A. If your vaginal secretion has an unusual or unpleasant smell or changes colour or if you feel itchy or sore, you may have a vaginal infection. You should go to a doctor or women's health centre because you may need treatment.

Some of the common infections include:
Gardnerella lives normally in the vagina, but can increase in number and cause problems. Symptoms include a greyish/green, watery discharge and an unpleasant smell. Treatment is by tablets and Aci-Jel cream to make the vagina more acidic.
Candida (Thrush) also lives in the vagina without causing problems. At certain times in your life, such as during menopause, pregnancy, illness, periods of stress or if you take antibiotics, the organisms may increase. Symptoms include a cheesy white discharge with an unu-

sual smell and a very itchy vagina that will get sore, because you have to scratch it all the time! Sexual intercourse will be painful. Treatment includes either vaginal creams or pessaries and tablets by mouth. Other helpful remedies include putting natural yoghurt or Aci-Jel cream in the vagina, or soaking a tampon in a weak solution of vinegar and warm water (one part vinegar to four parts warm water) and putting it in the vagina for 10 minutes morning and night. If you have a sexual partner, they should be treated at the same time, as the infection may be passed on during sexual contact.

Trichomoniasis can also be naturally occurring in the vagina or can be passed on during sexual contact. Symptoms are a frothy, thin, yellow discharge with an unpleasant smell. Treatment is by tablets and your sexual partner will also need to be treated.

Blood-stained discharge is common around menopause as a result of changes in your hormonal balance. However, you should always report any unusual bleeding to your doctor as it could be something more serious and need investigation. Any bleeding that occurs after menopause (after your periods have ceased) should be reported to your doctor as soon as possible.

To keep your vagina healthy:

- Wear cotton underpants, change them daily
- Don't wear underpants in bed (let it breathe!)

- Avoid tight jeans and pantyhose
- Never use perfumed talcs or deodorants
- Wipe toilet paper from front to back
- Eat a healthy, well-balanced diet
- Have regular sex, through intercourse or masturbation.

SMOKING – GIVE UP

Women who smoke often experience menopause a few years earlier than those who do not smoke. Nicotine may in fact decrease the secretion of hormones and alter the metabolism of sex-related hormones.

This can increase symptoms, such as hot flushes. Smokers may also lose more calcium from their bodies and increase their risk of osteoporosis.

You are probably aware of the other health risks connected with smoking, such as cancer, heart disease and lung problems. Mid-life is the time to stop smoking if you value your health. It may be a very difficult habit to break but help is available. You could try joining a stop-smoking programme, try hypnotherapy or acupuncture or just go it alone.

Chapter 6
Hormone Replacement: Blessing or Curse?

The most controversial aspect of menopause management is hormone replacement therapy (HRT). If you are totally confused, be reassured that you are not alone – many health professionals are also confused.

What are we to believe? Is taking artificial hormones for the rest of your life the answer for all your symptoms or should you just give it a miss?

WHAT IS HRT?

Hormone replacement therapy is the replacement of those hormones that are reduced after menopause. It is sometimes called ERT [estrogen (US spelling) or oestrogen therapy]. HRT is not the same as taking the oral contraceptive pill, which contains synthetic oestrogens and is much stronger. The oestrogens used in HRT are called natural oestrogens, because they are identical to the oestrogens in your body and are weaker than the synthetic ones. Unless a woman has had a hysterectomy, she will also be given progestogen, a synthetic form of progesterone, to reduce the risk of cancer of the lining of the uterus.

WHY THE DEBATE?

Hormone replacement treatment for menopause has been used widely since the early 1960s, particularly in the United States. Originally, oestrogen was given alone until researchers discovered a relationship with increased risk of cancer of the lining of the uterus. In the 1970s, progestogen (synthetic progesterone) was combined with the oestrogen to reduce this risk. In Britain only around 8 per cent of women take hormone replacement therapy and not many go on taking it for more than 6 months.

One reason why women stop taking HRT is because doctors do not always explain the possible side effects which can occur for the first few months, such as sore breasts, leg cramps, nausea, headaches and irregular bleeding.

In the United States, approximately 30–40 per cent of women take HRT. Recent US research indicates that those women who have been on HRT for more than 15 years have a longer life-expectancy and a lower risk of death from causes such as cancer.

The long-term benefits of HRT appear to be a reduced risk of heart disease, stroke and osteoporosis. The short-term benefits include relief from physical symptoms, such as hot flushes, dry vagina, bladder problems and insomnia.

The big question about HRT is whether or not it increases the risk of breast cancer. So far, studies have not proved conclusive.

YOUR BONES, YOUR HORMONES AND . . .

The density of strength of your bones is usually set by the time you reach 30. If you grew up on a dairy farm, drank lots of milk and ate plenty of cheese and cream, you will probably have bones like concrete. This is because your diet was high in calcium which is important for maintaining strong bones.

Bones are made up of an outer part (cortical bone) and an inner part (trabecular bone). Trabecular bone looks a bit like honeycomb and is present in large amounts in your spine, hips and wrists. It is the part of your bones that is most affected by bone loss in later life. From the age of about 30, you will start to lose small amounts of both types of bone. After menopause, the rate of this bone loss will increase, particularly in the first few years after your last period.

This acceleration in bone loss is caused by the reduced level of oestrogen in your body. Men also lose bone at an increased rate when they have low levels of testosterone. Thinning of bones is a part of growing old and, as a result, fractures or breaks in older people are quite common.

. . .OSTEOPOROSIS

Osteoporosis is a slow-moving and silent disease. More common in women than in men, it is a disease process resulting in a reduction of bone mass. Osteoporosis is caused by an excessive loss of calcium, collagen and other connective tissue from the bone.

The problem is compounded by the reduced ability of the body to make new bone after middle age. By the age of about 80, one in 4 women will have fractured their wrist, spine or hip as a result of osteoporosis.

The early signs of osteoporosis are:

- Loss of height
- Stooping of the spine
- Aches and pains in the bones.

Loss of oestrogen after menopause is the major cause of osteoporosis, but not the only one. Some of the other factors that will increase your risk of developing osteoporosis are:

- An early menopause (before 45)
- If you are fair skinned and thin
- If your mother, grandmother or sisters have osteoporosis
- If you use cortisone, antacids and some diuretics

- If at some time you did not menstruate regularly (did not have a period for more than 2 years)
- Because of anorexia or excessive exercise
- If your diet has been low in calcium and high in salt, protein, caffeine and fibre
- If you smoke or drink alcohol to excess
- If, as a child, you spent long periods in bed due to illness
- If you have a lack of vitamin D
- If you do not exercise.

ARE YOU AT RISK?

How many of these risk factors apply to you? If you think that you may be at risk of developing osteoporosis, then you should have a bone densitometry test. This simple and painless test measures the bone density in your spine, hips or wrist and determines your risk of developing osteoporosis. Ask your doctor about it.

The most effective way of preventing osteo-porosis after menopause is to take oestrogen. Not every woman will be at the same level of risk of developing osteoporosis, so weigh up <u>your</u> situation carefully before deciding whether or not to take HRT.

Other ways you can help to maintain heal-thier bones include: eating a well-balanced diet, rich in calcium; doing regular weight-bearing exercise, such as walking; reducing your alco-hol intake and stopping smoking.

THE IMPORTANCE OF CALCIUM

We have more calcium in our bodies than any
other mineral. Essential for strong bones and
teeth, it also plays an important role in the
functioning of our muscles, nerves, glands
and blood vessels. After menopause, you probably need around 1500 mg of calcium each day.
This may not be possible to achieve through
your diet alone. You would need to drink a litre

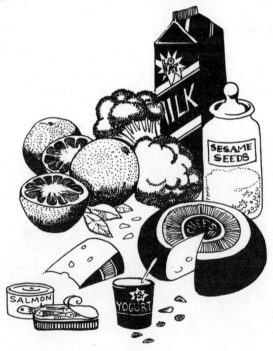

of milk each day to have an intake of 1000 mg of calcium. If you do drink milk, then it is better for your health to drink low-fat, calcium-enriched milk. Other good sources of calcium in the diet include: yoghurt; cheese; salmon; sardines; certain vegetables, such as broccoli, and fruit, such as oranges.

Supplements can increase your calcium intake but a few words of caution: don't take calcium supplements if you have a history of kidney stones, and high doses can cause constipation. If you take supplements, take them at night, before going to bed. This is the time when blood levels of calcium drop and you are more likely to lose calcium from your bones. Taking calcium alone will not prevent osteoporosis.

HEART DISEASE AND HORMONES

Women, pre-menopause, are less likely than men to suffer from cardiovascular disease. After menopause, changes in your cholesterol balance increases your risk of hardening and blockage of the arteries.

Recent research indicates that oestrogen offers women some protection from heart attacks and stroke by raising the level of HDL cholesterol (the goodies) and reducing the level of LDL cholesterol (the baddies).

Oestrogen can also act on the lining of the blood vessel walls, lessening the likelihood of cholesterol deposits and the resultant blockages.

You have lipoproteins in your blood that carry fat and cholesterol. There are two types: high density lipoproteins (HDL), that carry cholesterol away from the cells and tissues, and low density lipoproteins (LDL), that deliver the cholesterol to your organs and can deposit it in the walls of your arteries.

After menopause your total cholesterol and (LDL) cholesterol increases and so does your risk of cardiovascular disease.

You can help to reduce your total cholesterol level by:

- losing weight
- exercising
- lowering your intake of saturated fats, found in meats and whole-milk dairy products.

BREAST CANCER AND HORMONES

Many women are worried about taking HRT because of the risk of breast cancer. Some studies show a slightly increased risk of breast cancer, while others show a reduced risk. Recent studies indicate that if breast cancer develops in a woman taking HRT, it is more likely to be detected early by her doctor and may be a more slow-growing type of cancer. If you have had breast cancer, it is unlikely that your doctor would recommend HRT.

If you are worried about breast cancer or

have risk factors for breast cancer (see Chapter 8), discuss your worries in great detail with your doctor before deciding about HRT.

WHAT HAPPENS IF YOU CHOOSE HRT?

HRT is taken to relieve symptoms such as hot flushes, dry vagina, bladder problems and insomnia. It is also used in the prevention of osteoporosis and to reduce the risk of heart disease.

Q. *How do I take HRT?*
A. Hormones can be taken by: tablets, implants under the skin, injections, vaginal creams or pessaries and by skin patches. The most common method is by tablets. Each of these methods is described more fully later on.

The dosage is determined by your doctor and will vary with each woman. In the beginning, it may need to be adjusted to suit you, depending on how you respond. It is essential to have a thorough checkup by your doctor before you commence hormone replacement therapy. (See Chapter 8.)

Tablets: You will need to take an oestrogen tablet every day and a progestogen tablet, either every day or for 12–14 days of each month. If you have had a hysterectomy, you won't need to take the progestogen tablet. Progestogen is only given to stop the lining of your uterus from thickening, perhaps increasing your risk of cancer.

If you still have your uterus, then you will probably have a bleed each month. If this is very heavy or is a problem for you, your doctor can adjust the dose and schedule. Ideally, after being on the tablets for a while, you will not have a bleed at all. Even though you have bleeding, it is not like menstrual bleeding and it does not mean that you could become pregnant. There are a few different types of both oestrogen and progestogen tablets; you may find that some suit you better than others. The three most commonly used oestrogen tablets are Premarin, Hormonin and Progynova. The most commonly used progestogen tablets are Provera, Primolut-N or Micronor.

Implants: A small pellet is inserted under the skin by a doctor, using local anaesthetic. It only takes a few minutes. The implant can be put into your abdomen, thigh or buttock. There are three different strengths that last for an average of 2, 6 or 12 months.

The advantage of an implant is that you don't have to remember to take a pill every day. However, if you haven't had a hysterectomy, you will still need to take a progestogen tablet for 12 to 14 days each month to reduce the risk of cancer of the uterus.

The male hormone, testosterone, is sometimes also used as an implant for women who have a low libido or sex drive. This can cause side effects in some women, such as increased facial hair, weight gain and pimples.

Patches: A small, clear adhesive patch containing oestrogen is placed on the skin twice a week. Patches come in three different strengths and are usually put on the buttock or lower back. You should put it on a different site each time. In hot climates, some women can develop a rash and the patches can fall off in the bath or under the shower. If you have a uterus, you will need to take progestogen tablets in addition to using the patch.

Creams and pessaries: Oestrogen can be taken by inserting cream or special tablets into your vagina. These are often used by women who have no symptoms other than a dry vagina or bladder problems. Only a small amount of cream is usually necessary. If you have a uterus and use this method for a long time, you will need to take progestogen as well, for 12–14 days each month, to reduce the risk of cancer of the uterus. Pessaries, or tablets, are less messy and are preferred by some women.

Q. *When do I stop HRT?*
A. You can stop taking HRT at any time, but it is best not to stop suddenly. You should cut down slowly and see what happens. If you have been taking HRT for symptoms, such as hot flushes, dry vagina, insomnia or bladder problems, and your symptoms return, then you will probably want to start again.

To prevent osteoporosis and reduce your risk of heart disease, you may choose to continue

HRT for life. If you are going to have an operation in hospital, stop taking HRT 6 weeks beforehand to reduce the risks of blood-clotting.

Advantages	Disadvantages
Relief of:	Possible:
hot flushes	bleeding
vaginal problems	nausea, headaches
bladder problems	sore breasts
mood changes due to	fluid retention
your symptoms	bloated feeling
insomnia	weight gain
	leg cramps
	increased blood
	pressure
Prevention of osteoporosis	
Protection from:	
heart disease	
cancer of the uterus	Possible slight
(with progestogens)	increase in risk of
cancer of the ovary	breast cancer

Use this table to help you weigh up the factors which may be involved in your decision about using HRT.

Q. *HRT – is it for me?*
A. Some women should not take HRT for medical reasons. If you have severe liver

disease, a history of breast or uterine cancer, high blood pressure or any undiagnosed vaginal bleeding, then HRT is not recommended. Other conditions, such as diabetes, fibroids, gall-bladder disease or recent blood clots, require careful assessment by your doctor.

Weigh up the benefits and risks for yourself, before making a decision about HRT. Remember, it is *your* decision.

Some of the things that may influence your decision are:

- Possible risks or benefits to your health
- Your symptoms and how they affect you
- Your beliefs about natural versus artificial therapies.

There are many women who say that HRT has changed their life and they feel wonderful. Other women complain of side effects and worry about the unknown risks. Whatever you decide about HRT, after carefully weighing up all the pros and cons and discussing it with your doctor, your decision will be the right one for you.

Chapter 7
When Your Body Lets You Down

BLEEDING AFTER MENOPAUSE

If you are on hormone replacement treatment, then, depending on what dosage and combination of hormones you are taking, you will probably have some periodic bleeding. If you are not taking hormones and you have ceased to menstruate, then report any vaginal bleeding to your doctor as soon as possible. Your doctor will examine you thoroughly and will probably order tests, such as blood tests, an ultrasound scan, a curette (D&C) or a biopsy of the lining of your womb. Sometimes a hysteroscopy or laparoscopy might be necessary. In the first procedure, a telescope is passed through the vagina to look inside your womb. In the second, the doctor passes a telescope through your navel to have a look inside your pelvis. This is done under anaesthetic.

Bleeding after menopause can be caused by

hormonal changes, fibroids, polyps, blood disorders, infection, damage to the vagina during intercourse and, less commonly, cancer of the uterus or cervix.

FIBROIDS

These are the most common tumours found in women, occurring in about 20 per cent of women over the age of 30. They are rarely malignant (cancerous) and can grow in the wall of the uterus, under the lining or on the outer surface.

The following symptoms may indicate fibroids:

- Your periods may become very heavy, particularly on the second or third day of bleeding
- Your periods may become more painful and you may also notice pressure on your bladder or bowel
- If the fibroid is large, you may notice some discomfort during orgasm, when the uterus contracts.

Fibroids are less common in women who have had a number of children, who are of slight build and who do not smoke. After menopause, fibroids often shrink in size, but can grow again with hormone replacement treatment.

Small fibroids that are not causing problems are not usually removed, especially in older women. However, if they are large or they are causing symptoms, then a hysterectomy (removal of the uterus) or myomectomy (removal of the fibroid only) are often performed.

HYSTERECTOMY

Many women are confused about the relationship between hysterectomy and menopause. Hysterectomy does not result in menopause, unless the ovaries are removed as well as the uterus. If the ovaries are left, natural menopause will occur at the genetically determined time. Following hysterectomy, the ovaries sometimes cease to function temporarily; this is due to damage to their blood supply during surgery. Hot flushes after hysterectomy are usually only temporary. If they continue and are causing problems, they can be treated with hormone replacement therapy.

A hysterectomy is a major operation, performed under a general anaesthetic, either through an incision in the lower abdomen or through the vagina. Reasons for having a hysterectomy include:

- Heavy bleeding
- Fibroids
- Endometriosis
- Chronic pelvic disease
- Cancer of the uterus, cervix, ovaries
- Prolapse of the uterus.

Talk to your doctor about the pluses and

minuses before making the decision to have a hysterectomy. Explore the alternative treatments that are available.

If you have cancer, a hysterectomy may be necessary to save your life. The decision to have your healthy ovaries removed, if you do not have cancer and if you have not yet gone through menopause, is a more difficult one. If you do decide to have your ovaries removed, then you will experience sudden, surgical menopause and symptoms may begin within a week or two of the operation. These symptoms can be treated with hormone replacement therapy.

Endometrial ablation is a new surgical technique that may eventually eliminate the need for hysterectomy in cases of very heavy bleeding. It involves burning the lining of the uterus either with laser or an electrical current. After this operation, as with hysterectomy, a woman can no longer have children. Endometrial ablation requires a general anaesthetic and is carried out through a small telescope, inserted into the uterus from the vagina. You will only need to stay in hospital for a day or so.

SORE BREASTS

Some women occasionally have very painful, tender breasts. This can be due to hormonal changes and is sometimes referred to as mammary dysplasia, fibroadenosis or mastitis.

It is extremely important for you to examine your breasts regularly, in order to detect any abnormality, such as a lump. (See Chapter 8.)

If you have sore breasts, here's what you can do to help:

- If your breasts are large, make sure you have a well-fitting cotton bra; a good bra is very important as you grow older.

- If you are taking hormone replacement therapy, talk with your doctor about reducing your dose or alternative ways of taking your oestrogen.

- Reduce your salt intake – too much salt can cause fluid retention.

- Reduce your caffeine intake by reducing your consumption of coffee, tea, chocolate, cocoa and cola drinks. Switch to herbal teas, or decaffeinated coffee. If you are used to large amounts of caffeine each day, reduce it slowly to avoid withdrawal symptoms, such as severe headaches.

- Vitamin B1 (Thiamine) tablets can be bought at any chemist or health food store. Try taking 50 mg two or three times a day for at least three months. Vitamin B1 is also plentiful in foods such as peas, beans, nuts, fortified cereals, fruit and meat.

- Vitamin B6 (Pyridoxine) is a natural diuretic which helps relieve fluid retention. Try taking 50 mg a day after meals. You can obtain other natural diuretics in foods, such as celery, parsley, cucumber, watercress and dandelion tea.

PROLAPSE

Your pelvic organs are supported by muscles and ligaments which can become weakened following childbirth, lack of oestrogen and ageing. A prolapse occurs when your uterus, bladder or bowel fall down into the vagina because of weakened muscles.

BLADDER & UTERUS NORMAL

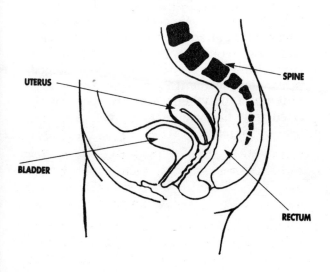

BLADDER & UTERUS
AFTER PROLAPSE

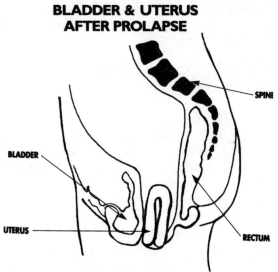

If you have a chronic cough, constipation or are overweight and have weak pelvic muscles as well, then you may be at risk. A prolapse usually requires surgery to repair the damaged muscles and ligaments, or a hysterectomy. Sometimes a polythene ring, or pessary, is inserted into the vagina to provide support, instead of surgery.

Chapter 8
Don't Put Up with Second Best

What can you expect at your age? Too often, older women are fobbed off by their doctors with insensitive comments, such as this. Well, don't put up with it. You should expect to be treated with respect, be listened to and have your concerns acknowledged. You have a right to high-quality health care and to be fully informed about the potential risks and benefits of any treatment.

Any alternative treatments should be outlined. The more you learn about menopause, whether by reading, attending a menopause education course or seminar or simply by talking with other women, the easier it will be to make informed decisions. After that, you may have to educate your doctor!

Q. *What should I look for in a doctor?*
A. Finding the right doctor can be a real challenge. Some doctors can communicate much better with their patients than others. Try to find one who:

- Has time to listen to you
- Is interested in you as a person
- Has a positive attitude to older women
- Has sufficient up-to-date knowledge
- Is prepared to refer you for specialist care, if necessary.

If you are not happy with your doctor, changing to another one under the NHS system may not be easy. If you would like to be able to talk to someone other than your doctor about menopause and how you are feeling, a visit to a Family Planning Clinic or Well Women's Clinic would be helpful. Staff at these centres are specially trained in all aspects of women's health and have access to the latest information about menopause.

You will also find that they are interested in you as a person, not just as a condition to be treated. They will be able to discuss a wide range of available choices with you.

ASKING THE RIGHT QUESTIONS

Communication is a two-way process. Your doctor can only respond to the information you give about yourself. It is important to describe clearly and accurately what you are experiencing. Keep a written record of your symptoms, describing what you experience. Note when and how often your symptoms occur.

Make a list of the questions you want to ask. How often do you remember all the things you meant to ask about <u>after</u> you leave the doctor's surgery.

Examples of the type of questions you may want to ask, include:

- Are my symptoms due to menopause?
- What treatments are available for these symptoms?
- What are the risks and benefits of the treatment?
- How does this treatment work?
- How long will I need to take it?
- What are the possible side effects?
- How much does it cost?
- What are my alternatives?
- What check ups should I have first?
- How often should I come back and why?
- Should I be referred to a specialist?

GETTING THE RIGHT ANSWERS

Many people have unrealistic expectations of their doctor. They sometimes expect an instant diagnosis, a quick fix and a miracle pill. The reality is very different. There are diseases and disorders that can be overlooked and mistakenly dismissed as being due to menopause. It is important to have a thorough check up, including any appropriate tests, before commencing any medical treatment. These may take some time, so be patient.

NECESSARY CHECK UPS

It is essential for the doctor to take a good medical history to find out all about you, your family and any relevant medical or social information.

You should have a physical examination including such things as: blood pressure test, breast examination, internal pelvic examination, cervical smear and feeling your abdomen. Blood tests to check your hormone and cholesterol levels should be done. You should also have a mammogram, a special breast screening X-ray. There are special tests that can determine your calcium levels and the condition of your bones. These tests can be expensive, but will help the doctor to assess your risk of osteoporosis, especially if you are undecided about hormone replacement treatment. It is important to see your doctor regularly, especially if you are on HRT, to monitor your treatment and dosages and to check on your general health.

CERVICAL SMEARS

All women who have ever had sexual intercourse should have regular cervical smears. A cervical smear is a simple screening test, which is usually performed every 3 years. The test can detect early changes in the cells of the cervix, which may progress to a more serious precancerous or cancerous form, if left untreated.

Q. *How is it done?*
A. A cervical smear takes only a few minutes and should cause little or no discomfort. A metal instrument, called a speculum, is inserted into the vagina to hold the vaginal walls apart gently. Some of the loose cells are wiped from around the small opening in the cervix, which is the part of the uterus that protrudes into the vagina. The cells are then placed on a glass slide and sent to a pathologist for examination. You should also have an internal pelvic examination and a breast check at the same time as the smear is done.

If you are not taking hormone replacement therapy, it may be difficult to take an adequate sample of cells from your cervix, after menopause. Your doctor may recommend that you take oestrogen for one week before your smear – either in the form of tablets or by placing pessaries or cream into your vagina. You will be advised not to insert the cream on the night before your smear.

Q. *What if I've had a hysterectomy?*
A. If you have had a hysterectomy, you will no longer have a cervix. Many years ago, the cervix was sometimes left in place during a hysterectomy, but this is not usually the case these days. If your hysterectomy was performed because of cancer, you will need to have regular

smears taken from the upper end of your vagina, as well as a pelvic examination and breast check. If your hysterectomy was not performed because of cancer, then a vaginal smear may only be necessary every few years. You will still need to have a regular pelvic examination, particularly if you still have your ovaries, and a breast check.

Q. *What if something's wrong?*
A. An abnormal smear can mean that you have an infection or that there are abnormal changes in the cells of your cervix. A further examination of these cells may be necessary. This is usually done with a microscope, called a colposcope, placed at the entrance to the vagina. Treatment of abnormal cells is not always necessary, but if it is required, the cells may be removed by laser, freezing, burning or biopsy.

BREAST SELF-EXAMINATION – MAKE IT A HABIT

The risk of developing breast cancer before the age of 75 is about one in 15. Those who are at greater risk of developing breast cancer are women who:

- Are over 40
- Have a mother or sister with breast cancer
- Have already had breast cancer in one breast
- Have never had a child
- Had their first child after the age of 30.

By regularly examining your own breasts, you will become familiar with how they normally feel and will be more likely to detect any changes, such as a lump or other irregularities. You should examine your breasts once a month, on the first day after the end of a period. If you no longer have periods, then mark the same day on your calendar each month to help you to remember.

Q. *How do I do it?*
A. There are two important aspects to breast self-examination – looking at your breasts and feeling them.

Looking

- Stand in front of a well-lit mirror. Look at your breasts for signs of dimpling or puckering of the skin or a difference in the appearance of your nipple.

- Keep looking as you hold your hands down at your side

- Raise your arms above your head

- Put your hands on your hips, press down and tighten your chest muscles

- Lean slightly forward, particularly if you have large breasts.

Feeling

You can do this under the shower or while lying down. In the shower, use your wet, soapy hands to examine your breasts.

In the shower

- Put one hand behind your head. With the other hand, using the flat of your fingers together, not your fingertips, gently move them all over your breast.

- Use a circular motion, making sure that you cover one segment at a time.

- Cover the area up to and including your armpit, as well as the nipple.

- Repeat for the other breast.

Lying down

You may find this easier if you have larger breasts.

- Put a pillow under one shoulder and place that hand behind your head.

- Using the flat of your fingers, cover the whole breast with gentle, circular motions, either in segments or in expanding circles. Don't forget the armpit area or the nipple.

If you are unsure of how to examine your breasts, ask your doctor or nurse practitioner to show you when you have your next cervical smear. If you have a partner, ask them to check your breasts regularly as well.

Q. *When should I worry?*
A. See your doctor as soon as possible if you find any of the following:

- A lump or thickening of the breast or nipple
- Change in the size or shape of the breast or nipple
- Any dimpling of the skin
- Discharge from the nipple
- Rash on the nipple
- Lump in your armpit.

If your doctor does not appear worried about it, but you are, get a second opinion.

Q. *What's a mammogram?*
A. This is a special breast X-ray that is used for screening as well as diagnosis. The breast is flattened on a special machine to allow a clearer picture to be taken. It can be quite uncomfortable, but only takes a few minutes.

All women over 40 should have regular mammograms, annual breast checks and examine their own breasts once a month.

Glossary

Adrenal Glands: Small glands above the kidneys which secrete sex hormones, adrenalin and cortisone.

Androgens: Male sex hormones secreted by the testes, adrenal glands and, in small amounts, by the ovaries.

Antioxidants: Substances that protect the body from damage.

Artificial Menopause: Cessation of periods after surgical removal of the ovaries or following radiation.

Biopsy: Removal and examination of tissue from the body to make a diagnosis.

Calcium: A mineral that is essential to prevent osteoporosis.

Cancer: An abnormal growth of cells, which destroy organs and can cause death.

Cardiovascular Disease: Any disease that affects blood circulation and oxygen supply to the body.

Cervical Smear: A regular screening test to detect any changes in the cells of the cervix.

Cervix: Neck of the uterus that protrudes into the vagina.

Cholesterol: Fatty substance normally present in the body. Too much can cause deposits in the blood vessels, increasing the risk of heart attacks.

Climacteric: The years before and after the last menstrual period.

Clitoris: Primary female organ of sexual arousal.

Clonidine: A drug that is sometimes used to control hot flushes.

Collagen: Protein which forms part of the tissues, supporting skin, bones and cartilage.

Colposcopy: A medical procedure which uses an instrument called a colposcope to look for abnormal cells around the cervix.

Condom: Latex sheath, placed on the erect penis before intercourse, to prevent sperm entering the vagina and to protect against sexually transmitted diseases.

Contraception: Birth control.

Cortical Bone: The outer layer of bone.

Curette: An instrument used to scrape the lining of the uterus.

Depo Provera: An injectable, long-acting progestogen that can be used as a contraceptive.

Diaphragm: A contraceptive latex dome that covers the cervix.

Dowager's Hump: Curving of the upper spine caused by compression of the vertebrae.

Endocrine Glands: Ductless glands that secrete hormones into the bloodstream and affect the organs of the body.

Endometrial Ablation: A surgical procedure that burns the lining of the uterus with laser or electric current.

Endometriosis: A condition in which the lining of the uterus grows outside it, on the ovaries, fallopian tubes and pelvic ligaments.

Endometrium: The lining of the uterus, shed during menstruation.

Ethinyl Oestradiol: A synthetic form of oestrogen.

Fatty Acids: Found in the diet, necessary for body cells.

Fallopian Tubes: Tubes connected to each side of the uterus, in which fertilisation occurs.

Fibroids: Non-cancerous growths, found in or on the uterus.

Follicle: Egg-forming cells in the ovaries.

Follicle Stimulating Hormone (FSH): A hormone secreted by the pituitary gland. It stimulates the egg cells in the ovary to grow and produce oestrogen.

Formication: A sensation of ants crawling under the skin. One of the symptoms of menopause.

Fracture: A break in a bone.

Genital Organs: The sexual organs.

Gynaecologist: A doctor who specialises in the treatment of conditions of the female reproductive system.

HDL Cholesterol: High density lipoprotein cholesterol, the 'good' cholesterol, has a protective effect in regard to heart disease.

Hormone: A chemical substance secreted by an endocrine gland, that affects other organs.

Hormone Replacement Therapy (HRT): The use of hormones to treat the symptoms of menopause.

Hot Flush: A sensation of intense heat, usually accompanied by reddening of the skin and perspiration.

HRT: Hormone replacement therapy.

Hypertension: High blood pressure.

Hypothalamus: An area of the brain which controls the reproductive centres in women and men, and other body functions.

Hysterectomy: Removal of the uterus.

Implant: A small device inserted under the skin to deliver hormones.

Incontinence: The inability to control bladder or bowel function.

Insomnia: The inability to sleep.

IUD: Intrauterine contraceptive device.

Labia: The lips that surround the entrance to the vagina.

LDL Cholesterol: Low density lipoprotein cholesterol.

Libido: Sex drive.

Lipoproteins: Proteins in the blood that carry lipids.

Luteinising Hormone (LH): A hormone that triggers ovulation.

Mammogram: A special breast X-ray.

Mastectomy: Surgical removal of the breast.

Masturbation: Self-pleasuring, stimulation of the body to produce orgasm.

Menopause: A woman's last menstrual period.

Menstruation: Cyclic bleeding and shedding of the lining of the uterus.

Metabolism: A combination of chemical and physical changes in the body, necessary to convert food for energy.

Oestradiol: A potent natural oestrogen.

Oestrogen: The female sex hormone, produced

in the ovaries.

Oestrone: A natural oestrogen.

Oral Contraceptive: Birth control pill.

Orgasm: Sexual climax.

Osteoporosis: Bone loss resulting in weak bones.

Ovaries: Female sex glands which produce hormones and eggs.

Ovum: An egg produced by the ovary.

Palpitations: Irregular or rapid heart beat.

Peak Bone Mass: Maximum amount of bone in the skeleton, usually set by the age of 20 or 30.

Pelvic Floor Muscles: Support for the organs of the pelvis.

Perimenopause: Period of time around the menopause.

Pituitary Gland: The gland at base of brain which controls other glands in the body.

Polyp: A growth occurring in a body cavity.

Postmenopause: The time after a woman's last period.

Premature Menopause: When menopause occurs before the age of 40.

Premenopause: The time before menopause.

Premenstrual Syndrome (PMS): The physical and emotional symptoms associated with the menstrual cycle.

Progestogen: A synthetic progesterone.

Vertebrae: Bone segments of the spine.

Vitamins: Naturally occurring substances vital to life.

Vulva: Female external genital organs.

Womb: The uterus.

Helpful Addresses

There are a number of organisations that offer advice and support specifically for women who are experiencing problems because of the menopause. The Family Planning Association in London will be able to give you a contact in your own area, as will the Marie Stopes Clinics.

Elizabeth Garrett Anderson Hospital
144 Euston Road
London
NW1 2AP
(0171) 387 2501 ext. 225
(Self-referral clinic for all women. Offers a range of services to those experiencing the menopause.)

Family Planning Association
27–35 Mortimer Street
London
(0171) 636 7866

Hysterectomy Support Group
11 Henryson Road
London
SE4
(0171) 690 5987

Marie Stopes Clinics
Marie Stopes House
108 Whitfield Street
London
W1P 6BE
(0171) 388 0662

Midlife Matters
32 Gwynne Road
Parkstone
Poole
Dorset
BH12 1AS
(0202) 735287
(Self-help group, willing to help with PMS, hysterectomy counselling, etc.)

Women's Health Concern
83 Earls Court Road
London
W8 6EF
(0181) 556 1966

ROBINSON FAMILY HEALTH

All your health questions answered in a way
you really understand.

Titles available from booksellers or direct from
Robinson include:

Arthritis: What *Really* Works
Dava Sobel & Arthur C. Klein
1–85487–290–7   £7.99

Asthma
Megan Gressor
1–85487–386–5   £2.99

Bad Backs: A Self-Help Guide
Leila Henderson
1–85487–388–1   £2.99

Bulimia Nervosa: A Guide to Recovery
Dr Peter Cooper
1–85487–171–4   £5.99

Headaches: Relief at Last
Megan Gressor
1–85487–391–1   £2.99

Let's Get Things Moving: Overcoming Constipation
Pauline Chiarelli and Sue Markwell
1–85487–389–X   £2.99

Massage for Common Ailments
Penny Rich
Illustrated in full colour
1–85487–315–6   £4.99

Menopause Made Easy
Kendra Sundquist
1–85487–383–0   £2.99

Pregnancy and Birth
Kerrie Lee
1–85487–390–3   £2.99

Overcoming IBS
Dr Christine P. Dancey & Susan Backhouse
1–85487–175–7   £5.99

Practical Aromatherapy
Penny Rich
Illustrated in full colour
1–85487–315–6   £4.99

The Recovery Book: A Self-Help Guide for Recovering Alcoholics, Addicts and Their Families
Al J. Mooney, Arlene Eisenberg & Howard Eisenberg
1–85487–292–3   £9.99

Women's Waterworks
Pauline Chiarelli
1–85487–382–2   £2.99

You *Can* Beat Period Pain
Liz Kelly
1–85487–381–4   £2.99

How to Order

To order a book, please send a cheque (made out to Robinson Publishing Ltd) or postal order to the address below, adding 50p per title for postage and packing. Send to: **Family Health, Robinson Publishing Ltd, 7 Kensington Church Court, London W8 4SP.**

While this information was correct at the time of going to press, details may change without notice.